Author Terry L. Ware Sr. Presents:

PoEtIc XpReSsIoNs: Vol 3, *Variations of Anxiety Disorders*

The Xpressions Group III

General Information

PoEtIc XpReSsIoNs: Vol 3, Variations of Anxiety Disorders
The Xpressions Group III

All Rights Reserved. No part of this publication may be reproduced, stored in a retrieval system, or transmitted, in any form or in any means – by electronic, mechanical, photocopying, recording or otherwise – without prior written permission of the "Material Owner" or its Representative **B.O.S.S. Publishing, LLC**. Any such violation infringes upon the Creative and Intellectual Property of the Owner pursuant to International and Federal Copyright Law. Any queries pertaining to this "Collection" should be addressed to Publisher of Record.

Copyright © 2021:
The Xpressions Group III

Cover Design: ***B.O.S.S. Publishing- Terry L. Ware Sr.***

Publisher: ***B.O.S.S. Publishing***

Editor: ***Terry L. Ware Sr.***

ISBN: ***978-0-9988341-9-1***

1. ***Poetry*** 2. ***Mental Health*** 3. ***Anthology*** 4. ***Anxiety***

3rd Edition

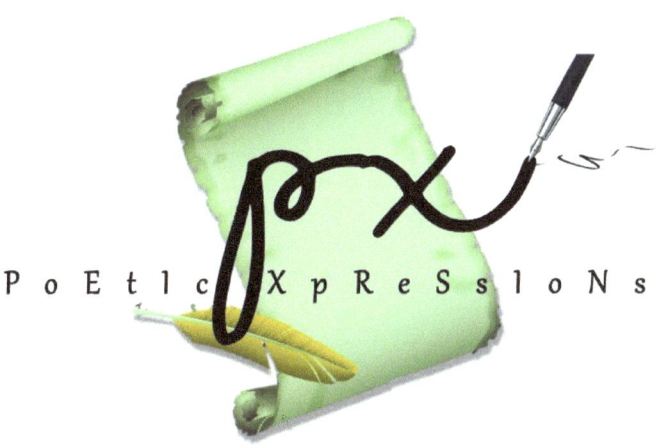
PoEtIc XpReSsIoNs

Dedication

PoEtIc XpReSsIoNs: Vol 3 is dedicated to those that have or may be dealing with any kind of Anxiety. You are not DEFEATED! You will not LOSE! May the God of Peace and Comfort propel you into your complete deliverance.

Foreword

This Book is a True-life changing Statement of real-life facts & stories of trails & Triumphs. A MUST READ!!!

Kelvin "K Chill" Harris
CEO The ATL Actors Awards
CEO Chillzone Entertainment

Table of Contents

Dedication..iii
Foreword...iv

How Can I Breathe...1
   By: Terry L. Ware Sr

Chapter 1

Panic Disorder...4

   The Constant Unknown- Tiffany S. Hooks..........5
   Reality Is- LaMia Pierce..7
   Lost: 38 Years Old And Still Searching-
   Maya C. Houston...13
   The Art Of Patience- Keiona McGhee.................18

Chapter 2

Social Anxiety Disorder.............................20

   Slumber Is My Refuge- Maya C. Houston...........21
   Release- Keiona McGhee......................................24
   Monsters- LaMia Pierce..25
   Racing Of The Mind- Tiffany S. Hooks...............29

Chapter 3

Specific Phobias Disorder..................31

The Root Of It All- LaMia Pierce........................32
You're Not Alone- Tiffany S. Hooks....................35
Wandering- Keiona McGhee..............................38
Dis-Ease- Maya C. Houston.............................40

Chapter 4

Generalized Anxiety Disorder..............................42

Altered Reality- Keiona McGhee.........................43
GAD- Maya C. Houston..................................44
Determined- Tiffany S. Hooks..........................48
Her Brokenness- LaMia Pierce..........................50

Epilogue

About the Poets.................................63

Tiffany S. Hooks......................................64
LaMia Pierce..67
Keiona McGhee...70
Maya C. Houston.......................................71

Symptoms & Causes..............................74

HELP HOTLINES..................................76

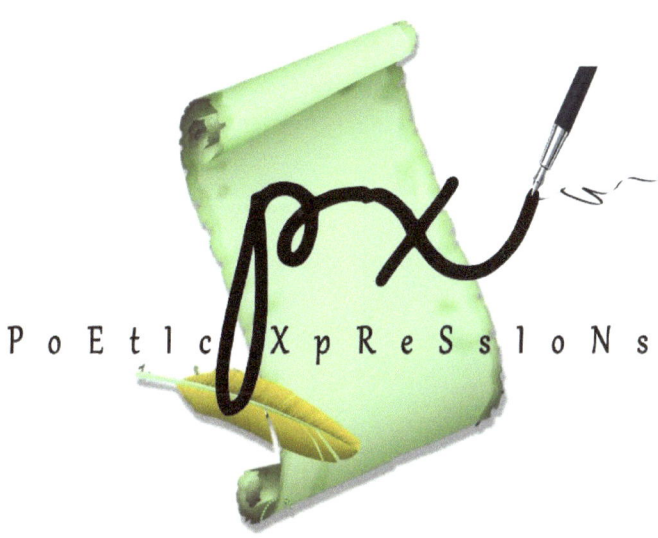

Author Terry L. Ware Sr. Presents:

PoEtIc XpReSsIoNs: Vol 3, Variations of Anxiety Disorders

The Xpressions Group III

How Can I Breathe
By: Terry L Ware Sr.

Where do I begin

The feeling of uneasiness seems to be the trend

Sleepless nights leads to limited sight

Staying calm is unfathomable

So still moments becomes my fight

But I'm alive, right

Early mornings

Late nights

Hands filled with sweat

Followed by the numbness of my toes

But you say

BREATHE

HOW

Heart pumping fast

A lifetime it seems to last

It's the air I'm struggling to grasp

But you say

BREATHE

HOW

Fluids being indulged

Yet

Consumed by the dryness of my mouth

Mind racing

Thoughts of the unknown become stronger and stronger

I endeavor to be free

Yet

These emotions enslave me

Is this room spinning

Or is it just me

But you say

BREATHE

HOW

Chapter 1
Panic Disorder

The Constant Unknown
By: Tiffany S. Hooks

Shhhh... Shhhh...

Pause

Inhale

Exhale

I can't stop you

Why are you here again

What did I do to warrant this sudden intrusion from you

The sun no longer shines upon me as the gray clouds come in

The joy is overcome with darkness

Why

Why

Did my smile frighten you

Did my peace unravel you

Is that why you have come to attack me yet again

Shhhh... Shhhh...

As my tears fall and my heart races

I will inhale and exhale the dread that's upon me

Will you ever cease and leave me in peace

Reality Is
By: LaMia Pierce

In the wake of this pandemic

She was faced with the fear

Fear that ripped at her heart

Faced stained with tears

Faced with the reality

The world as she has known it

Was now smeared with fears

There she stood with her heart in her knees

Paralyzed with emotions

Unsure of how to feel

Unsure of how to breathe

Catch her breath

Variations of Anxiety Disorders

This pain throbbing

Stabbing in her chest

Help she wanted to scream

But silence echoed thru her lips

She tried to walk

Nothing but motionless hips

No talk

No walk

No air to breathe

Just paralyzed with fear

This feels like the end just might be near

This can't be life

This can't be true

This can't be the new norm

She was determined to weather this storm

Run her race

Glide with grace

Wipe the tears from her face and her heart

The world was ready

So was she to play her part

At least so she thought

Her steps never hit the pavement

Of the front door

Yearning for more

To life

To reality

The panic set in

She sat by the window

Knowing this race she would not win

Variations of Anxiety Disorders

Maybe not today

But one day the fear will begin to dissipate

That will be the day

She looks fear in the eye

No more hiding behind the ugly disguise

Or the fake smiles

She suffered too long to not win the award for the winning part

She took her anxiety

Looked it right in the face

Said goodbye

Wiped the tears off her face

Proceeded to run with grace

As her mentality became clear

Her purpose did too

Sharing her story on mental health

Was her battle to save someone like you

To tell the story

Earn her crown

Tears falling never to weigh her down

She did it

I did it

We all played apart

Next time your heart beats

Know we are not far apart

I walked in your shoes

Now you are walking in mine

This friendship is forever

Sister friends from the heart…

I know your pain

Variations of Anxiety Disorders

I feel it to

Anxiety and panic

Looks like me

Looks like you

The beauty of it all is in the first step

I will see you at the finish line

Holding your spot so you can take your rightful place

Bold

Fierce

Unapologetically proud

No more fakeness just genuine smiles

Lost: 38 Years Old And Still Searching

By: Maya C. Houston

I found myself crying behind my bathroom door

For no apparent, immediate reason and for every thinkable reason one could imagine

I am living in an apartment with my daughter

Section 8 - Dirty walls - Dirty carpets

Low income and lots of skills in the land of opportunity

And every opportunity seems to be outside of my grasp

My daughter approaches the bathroom door

"Mommy – Malala's dad is not a Pashtun man"

I answered

He is Pashtun

The question is

"is he a traditional Pashtun man

Why or Why not"

Zion whispers outside the door softly

So frail and timid as if she was feeling

What I was desperately trying to hide

She sounded scared and uncertain

My eyes were as red as a whiskey filled vagabond at the corner of King and Huger St

My face a mess

Pressed up against the door

Taking hard deep breaths before I speak

Trying to regain the control I had lost and keep losing over and over again

With each new twist of each new day

The same twists I used to welcome with courage and a positive outlook

The same twists I used to contain in zones and categories of possible solutions now seems to be rushing me

Unleashed

Unorganized

Unable to be comprehended all at once

All the time

I am armed, out of sync and out of breath

As I hold on tightly to the bathroom sink

Slow quick breaths

Tears flowing

Quietly whimpering and searching for answers at my age

Variations of Anxiety Disorders

I am lost

I am moving forward and standing still

Trying to calm myself with each quick short breath

But the feeling of displacement discouragement and uncertainty only intensify

I want to get into the shower and begin to wash away some of this anxiety

But I cannot move

I need to move but I am stuck

Stuck at the sink

Stuck at 1885 Harper Drive

Stuck at earning $14,000 a year before taxes

Stuck at the register putting back the things I need

Just so I can afford ONLY the things I need

I am stuck on the phone with GA Power

Scana Energy

And AT&T

Searching for ways to decrease my bills

And make arrangements so I can keep my services from being disconnected

The woman on the other line while appearing to be human

Keeps giving me plastic responses and no solutions

She throws out policies and procedure and all I want are lights

I am 38

I am lost

I am searching

I feel so much darkness

all I want is some darn light

The Art Of Patience
By: Keiona McGhee

What is patience and how does it align with my spirit

Why is it that when I awake

My mind feels tired from running all night and staying awake

How do you enjoy your own company

And find peace within your voice

When your voice is all you hear

And your echoes begin to stare back at you

Self-resiliency

For I am alone for a reason

This is my season of isolation

I stand silent to reveal my purpose

I am alone building confidence

Just because I stand alone does not mean

I stand worthless

Chapter 2
Social Anxiety Disorder

Slumber Is My Refuge
By: Maya C. Houston

Persistent sadness shattering every chance of gladness when I am awake

Eating my feelings

Then looking forward to sleep sums up how hopeless my days have become

Slumber is my refuge

When I go there I do not feel

I sleep in hopes to heal

I cannot wait to dream

As my dreams offer an escape

In my dreams I am living the life I've always wanted

Variations of Anxiety Disorders

Haunted by so many imbalances when I am awake

My smile

My laughter

And my joy – all fake

Withdrawing from family and friends

Loss of interest in my favorite things

Fatigue seems to own me

Covered in clouds - type lonely

Wishing every good thing I desire would just hold me

But

They don't - so I sleep

Even the smallest of disappointments seem so huge

I don't rest when I sleep

But

I can't wait to go there because slumber is my refuge

Release
By: Keiona McGhee

I'm praying for a deep sleep

Slightly lighter than death

So wake me up when happiness arrives

And my thoughts aren't in control of me

And when my reality isn't such

Non- fiction to me.

Monsters
By: LaMia Pierce

My story isn't yours

Your story isn't mine

The monsters look the same

Or maybe it's the fear they leave behind

Fear and anxiety

To share the pain

The pain of a story

That leaves you mentally drained

Spiritually dead

Physically lame

With no one to blame

But the monsters that look the same

Variations of Anxiety Disorders

Looking at you was like looking at me

I wonder if you recognized

The pounding of my heart

As my body attempted to release

This anxiety

You see it

Because I see it too

Because the monsters look the same

Do you recall from childhood

The monsters under the bed

I used to believe they were all in my head

Until their hands slowly crept up my leg

The pounding of my heart

Here comes the hurting part

As my body attempts to release

This anxiety

The monsters are tearing me apart

My story isn't yours

Your story isn't mine

It just has the same narrative of the pain and panic

Left behind

Of the monsters that look the same

I understand now

Why your reflection resembles me

We share the same pain

That was the root of what they

Label Anxiety

Panic

Fear

Variations of Anxiety Disorders

Hurt

Tears

Pounding hearts

Clenched fist

Paralyzed stance

Caused by the monsters that look the same

Racing Of The Mind
By: Tiffany S. Hooks

Shhh

Inhale

Exhale

Inhale

Exhale

Is what I am attempting to do

As dread seems to invade me

Overpowering is this feeling

But I still try to walk boldly amongst the crowd.

Clammy is my skin

And my heart is racing

Yet no one notices it.

I am seconds from a full-blown anxiety attack

Leaving would be my best option

Pulse running faster than a raging bull

After seeing the color red

Helpless

Oppressed

Breathe

I closed my eyes

Inhale

Exhale

Inhale

Exhale

I survived again

Amongst the crowd

Chapter 3
Specific Phobias Disorder

Variations of Anxiety Disorders

The Root Of It All
By: LaMia Pierce

What is it

The Root of it all

The Beginning of the end

When my reality began to fall

Fall to the thoughts

That continuously clouded my thoughts

Looking back over childhood traumas

Thinking I had to be at fault

The root of it all

When my reality began to fall

To my heart beating so fast

Fingertips on the buttons

Just in case 911 was the next call

From the thoughts and the anguish

The guilt and the shame

From the depression

And the suicidal thoughts

That won't leave my brain

From the memories

That taunt me

Driving me insane

If I can catch my breath

Maybe I can utter my name

To the person who is watching me

Waiting for me to speak

But this silence is so loud

Its deafening me

The root of it all

When my reality began to fall

I went to the ledge

Ready to end it all

But

God sent an angel

And that Angel caught it all

Braced my brokenness

Which was the root of it all

You're Not Alone
By: Tiffany S. Hooks

Do they know how you truly feel inside

Do they know that you are living

Surrounded by darkness

Do they know that you cry almost every day

Do they know that your inner being is screaming

Do they know that all you want is a hug

Do they know that that smile upon your face isn't genuine

Do they know even though you're surrounded by others

You still feel ALONE

Do they know

Do they know

Would they call you crazy if you spoke your truth

Would they truly understand

Would it even matter

It matters to God how you are feeling

It matters to God how you are living

It matters to God because you are His child

It matters to God because He loves you unconditionally

You matter because He created you for a purpose

And regardless of the adversities you may face

He equipped you with everything you need to overcome

Trust the process and endure through

The battle it's worth the journey

YOU matter

Because even in the midst of the storm

You're NOT ALONE

Wandering

By: Keiona McGhee

They say the mind is a terrible thing to waste

But I feel as if mine is wasting me

I find myself under the spirit of doubt

I begin to question my being

And despise my existence

The weight of my struggles sits heavily

Upon my shoulders

The strength that I once thought I had

Has abandoned me on this road

That seems to be frequently traveled

Yet

No one stops by

As if they can't see me

Or hear my cries

Here I am

My spirit lies

And screams

As I lay on the cold ground

Strung out on life's woes

As I lay here and think

There is no way

This hell will ever deliver me

Variations of Anxiety Disorders

Dis-Ease
By: Maya C. Houston

Physical pain casted upon my body from the stresses in my brain

It is hard to concentrate on anything outside of what worries me most

Depression is the ghost that controls me these days

Not to mention the rapid weight gain

The way bread, cookies, cake and chocolate candy soothes me

I abuse food while food abuses me

Eating releases a happy chemical in my cranial space

That seems to level the imbalance brought on by sadness

Food feels like love

Betty Crocker's brownies are like warm chocolatey hugs

King's Hawaiian's sweet rolls make me feel sunny on the inside

But

Only for a moment does this sadness subside

Then guilt sets in because the dis-ase of the idea of this disease consuming me

Puts me right back into the space of total melancholy

Chapter 4
Generalized Anxiety Disorder

Altered Reality
By: Keiona McGhee

There's nothing more perplexed than being

Trapped in one's mind

In a false narrative

That only I believe in

And once I confess my truths

Others tell me I'm false

And come down on me

Harder than this world has

Variations of Anxiety Disorders

GAD

By: Maya C. Houston

When I went to bed last night everything was fine

I woke up this morning in a panic

There was this looming fear that hung heavy around my neck and sat firmly upon my chest

Gasping for breath and running through countless checklists in my mind for the thousandth time

I can't put my finger on it

A rush of frantic voices sounding off in my head like a million bells

Asking

Telling

Saying

And praying everything in every different direction all at the same time

Something is wrong

Is something wrong

No

Nothing is wrong

Something will be wrong soon though

Impending doom takes over

Inside eyes crying but the heavy fear that hangs around my neck won't let tears come outside

Outside of this mindset is where I'd rather be

Praying each second

Variations of Anxiety Disorders

Lord, please don't let this consume me

I push through each new breath and 60 seconds of defeating unseen disaster brings me closer to the belief

That even within the next 59 seconds

I may be able to feel safe after

I keep wondering where it's all coming from

Is it behind me

In front of me

Or within the broken/unhealed child inside of me

I will continue to fight this second by second and minute by minute

Because even one day at a time can be quite heavy

When you're a superhero who battles generalized anxiety

Determined

By: Tiffany S. Hooks

My chest is getting tighter

As I'm overwhelmed

With worry and sadness

I slowly began to inhale and exhale

To relax the tension in my chest

There's no relief and now my thoughts

Are running rapid within my head

I'm trying to visualize

A sunny day

With blue sky's

To counter the darkness I feel

Why

Why

Why did you choose to seek me

Have you not caused havoc in my life

You come and go at will

And no one truly understands this but I

Inhale and exhale again

There's no relief

Please

Please release me

I want to be free

Free from your surprise visits

Without consulting me

In due time you won't control me

Variations of Anxiety Disorders

Her Brokenness
By: LaMia Pierce

Her brokenness was the root

the root to it all

The panic attacks

the anxiety

the sleepless nights

the endless lovers she took in

to feel the emptiness

of the voids she felt within

Her first taste of love never came from her mother's touch

her father's hugs

grandma's pies

or Sunday dinners

Her foundation was rocky

memories clouded by rooms filled with gloom

Dark living rooms over polluted

with the smell of booze and cigarette smoke

A missing mother

A jailbird father

Alcoholic grandmother

Two-bedroom project

I'm painting a picture, is it becoming clear

Most of the anxiety and depression

many face stems from broken years

Of childhood memories

That cut like broken glass

Shattered into pieces

Variations of Anxiety Disorders

that can never be glued back together

No wonder broken girls grow into broken women

I'm painting a picture is it becoming clear

With anger

hate

low self esteem

Chasing broken dreams

With no means to an end

From the storm that rages

Between the pages of erased memories

From borrowed pages

From the story you create to escape

The memories of a childhood

that can't be erased

Yeah

I know

it is the story of most black girls

From the hood

Teen pregnancy

Drug dealer boyfriends

R. Kelly

oh yeah

I had a few of them

just different names

Still the adults knew the game

They turned a blind eye

it was their story too

same song different tune

Variations of Anxiety Disorders

I'm painting a picture is it becoming clear

No wonder generational curses become

passed on cycles

passing on the brokenness

Of childhood traumas

High school dropout

no sense of identity

life of drama

But

It's not played out on the big stage

With lights and cheers

or the I love you

That was the word she wanted to hear

Suffering from depression

Who are you going to tell

That these voices won't shut up

are you better off dead

Here it comes

another panic attack

She feels like she is dying

maybe that's her sigh of relief

From the brokenness

the memories

That keep stealing her life

But isn't that the job of a thief

Her brokenness was the root

the root to it all

The reason why she continued to crawl

Undefeated by circumstances

Broken and all

but she remember the one-time

God sent an angel to catch her

before the fall

I'm painting a picture is it become clear

The years

The tears

The fears

The pain

Unidentified female

what is her name

Mirrorless images

unrecognizable to see

The beauty behind the scars

that cut so deep

I remember it all

although I try not too

Brokenness was the foundation

that started it all

I'm painting a picture is it becoming clear

I came across this quote that resonated and spoke to my spirit

It said

"broken crayons still color"

Profound right

I suffered from depression

anxiety attacks

and suicidal thoughts for a very long time

and when I came across that quote

it made my spirit leap

Those words gave me hope

that I can still have a life

that is fulfilling and has meaning

My breakthrough from the pains of mental health issues

did not come from the traditional means of therapy and drugs

by no means am I opposed to those methods

Your healing is your responsibility

and the method that one takes down that path to healing

is also unique

for one's own individual journey

For me

I faced my demons head on and it took many years

Those demons looked like alcoholism

abusive relationships

and low self-esteem

I was living a life that did not match

the vision that I had in my head

of the way I pictured my life to be

or wanted it to be for that matter

and that was the root of my anxiety

I was not being true to myself

I was living a lie

and I started to believe that lie

until I forced it to be a living truth

The more I lived in the illusion

the more forceful the panic attacks would become

Being a religious/spiritual individual

I always believed in the power of prayer

that was the ultimate saving grace for me

I took years to recover

along with a lot of self-forgiveness and self-love

I had to be brutally honest with myself

I had to fight past the traumas

forgive my parents

acknowledge my shame and my pain

I had to promise myself to live my life authentically

unapologetic

within my personal truth

and now today I am finally free

If you or someone you know is suffering from any type of mental health crisis/issue please speak up and speak out, seek help I promise you that you are not alone. Mental health in the black community has been frowned upon for far too long

Strong people get help, that is what gives one strength, being unafraid. Often times it only takes one person to be the voice. I hope as you read my words my voice can break the chains of bondage that have you bond.

I told myself a few years back that I will be the voice for those afraid to speak and I am committed to standing on those words.

I've never told my story, I held onto it like it was a badge of honor, but that was yet another illusion. For me with each false facade I opened up the door for fear to creep in which in turn always lead to anxiety or panic attacks.

One thing for certain and two things for sure, our stories may differ but the pain we share is the same. So yes, I can relate to you and yes I feel and share in your pain.

There will come a time when the fear paralyzes you and you become overwhelmed and out of places to hide. I know because it happened to me too. I dug deep, I made a choice to do the inner work, heal my inner child, talk about the abuse, express the pain I felt and I decided I was not running anymore, no more hiding. I challenge you to do the same. There is a freedom that liberates you when you speak your truth. You deserve to be set free, I did it, you can do it!

It's time to be set free 🦋

Our demons keep chasing us as long as we continue to keep running~

I am LaMia Michele and I write from the heart~

Epilogue

About The Poets

Tiffany S. Hooks

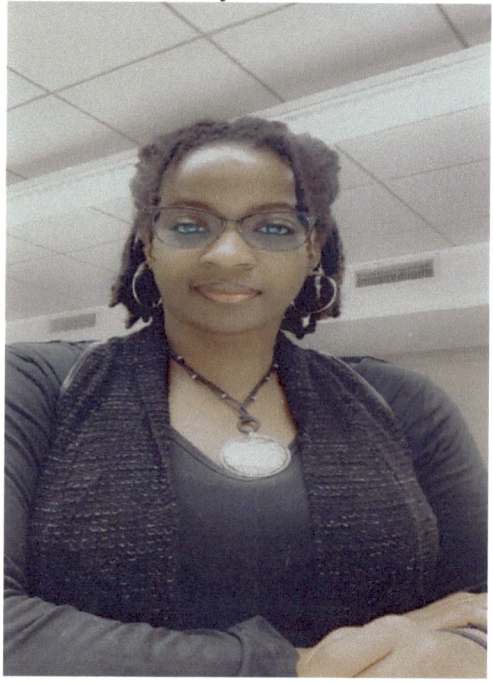

It is oftentimes through our pains through this journey called life that beauty blooms as shown through the journey of Author and Poetess, Tiffany S. Hooks.

This remarkable woman shows her readers through the power of words how she flourished and took the blows of life and was granted beauty for ashes.

Born in Douglas, Georgia, the second oldest daughter amongst seven siblings,

Tiffany found a best friend in herself through journaling and writing at a young age.

Not only is she an Author, a daughter, a sister and a mother to five amazing children: Jasmine E. Jordan, Thomas T. Hooks, Marcus K. Hooks, Maalik A. Hooks and the baby of the bunch Faatima M. Hooks, but she is also a seven-year breast cancer survivor.

While Tiffany wasn't prepared for the hand that life was sure to hand her, she was empowered by her circumstances and turned her pain into power.

This power is evident by the words she wrote in her self-published books, that can be found on Amazon.com.

Spiritual Journey to Perfection

Brokenness: Born, Broken & Rebuilt

Flourishing in Hope; Quotes to Give You Hope

You can keep in contact with Tiffany S. Hooks on her Instagram platform

@Mytruth_mywords.

Tiffany is also a certified life coach and is available for speaking engagements.

LaMia Pierce

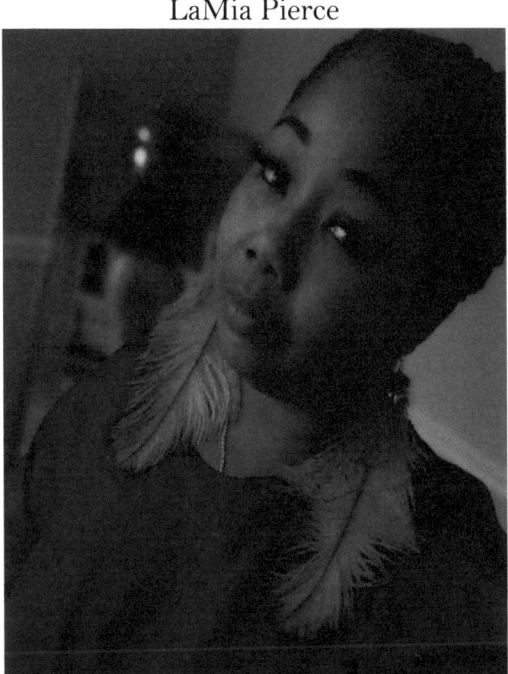

LaMia Michele was born and raised outside of Philadelphia, PA, in a small city that is packed with great history. That city is Chester, PA.

LaMia was brought up in the public school system where reading and writing became two of her favorite subjects. As she bloomed into young adulthood and now womanhood, those subjects became her favorite hobbies turned into passion and now into her healing!

While her style of writing is uniquely hers to own, there is one word that describes it perfectly, TRUTH.

LaMia Michele is a Poetess and what sets her apart and makes her unique is that she, in her words, "write's straight from my heart".

There is a scripture that comes to mind that embodies the words of this Poetess, "out of the abundance of her heart flows the issues of life". LaMia Michele's' writings tell her personal truth, her hurt and her pain, as well as the issues of depression that held her hostage for many, many years as she journeyed through life. Anxiety and panic attacks being an integral part of her story that paralyzed her for a massive amount of her life, yet she transmuted that energy into something magical.

Her route to healing came alongside her walk into her personal spiritual awakening. If LaMia had a message for those suffering from anxiety and panic attacks, she wants you the reader to know that there is beauty in pain and a blessing in the wound, get to the root of the problem so that your healing can begin.

In the words of this beauty undefined: "I LaMia Michele, promise you that you will do great things despite your anxiety, depression or whatever mental condition you may now face. I too once walked in your shoes and I am a living example of overcoming!"

LaMia Michele is a Certified Life Coach and first-time Published Author.

Her first book can be found on Amazon: "She Writes from the Heart"

For speaking engagements and to follow her journey you can also follow her on her social media platforms:

Facebook: @Mia Pierce

Instagram: @planted_seeds_444

Keiona McGhee

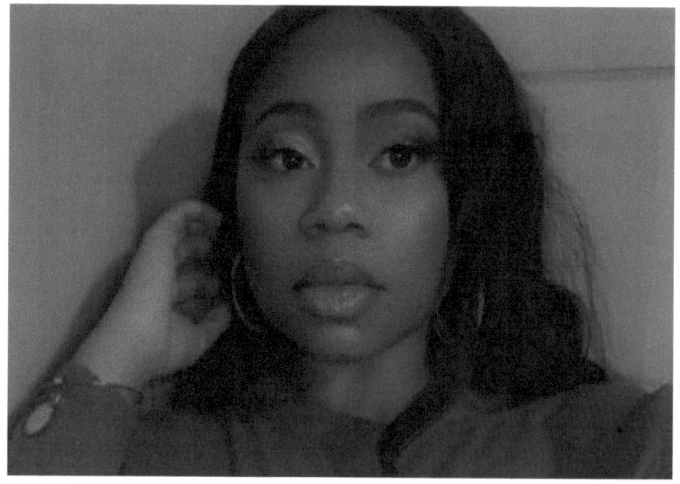

Keiona McGhee is 24 and feels ahead of her years which she says leaves her behind, yet actually in the perfect place.

Keiona is one of the sweetest spirits you will ever meet and loves almost everyone she is around.

In her own words, Keiona states:
"I pray these words I have been given, speaks to your mind, body, or your soul and comfort you. May you never feel alone".

Facebook: @Keiona McGhee

Instagram: @_bonita.k_

Maya C. Houston

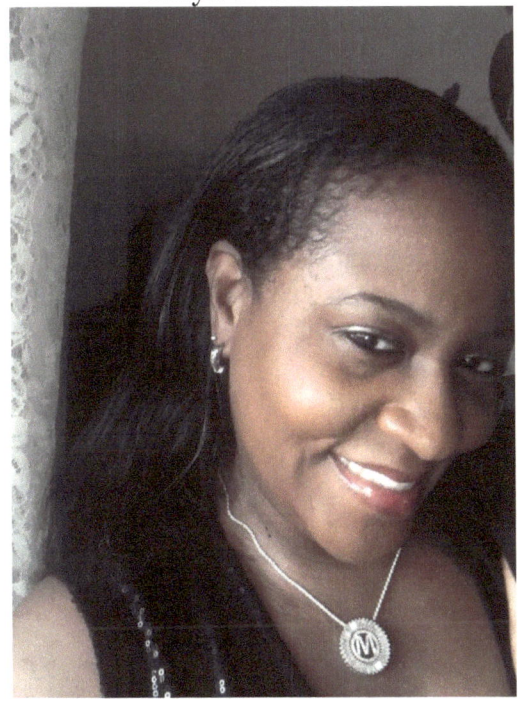

Maya C. Houston is a native of Charleston, S.C. Daughter to Truman and Mary T. Houston, she attended the local public schools and got her theatrical as well as public speaking start at New Israel Christian School. Under the tutelage of Marilyn Pyatt , Bishop S.K. Rembert, Julia Tyler and Martha Robinson, Ms. Morrison and a host of others, it was at New Israel that Maya began stage plays and speeches at the urging of her teacher Mrs. Marilyn Pyatt.

Maya moved on to attend James Simmons Elementary, Rivers Middle, and Middleton High for two years.

Due to the lack of social groups geared toward African American teenagers at Middleton, Maya and a group of her new friends founded Omega Phi Nu: Maya's friends elected her president. Omega Phi Nu was a sorority that started with 20 girls having a strong commitment to community service, self-love, and uplifting others. This was no easy task, it took protests, petitions, and supportive, vocal parents.

There came along a few other sororities and fraternities after the pioneering Omega Phi Nu and years later even after the original group graduated, O Phi Nu remained a thriving social force at Middleton High School. Maya helped start Omega Phi Nu and later moved on to Burke High School, where she graduated in 1995.

A move based on faith took Maya and her 1-year-old daughter, (Zion) to Atlanta Georgia. She attended Dental Assisting

School in Morrow GA., graduated and worked as a dental assistant while she completed a B.A. in Theatre (Clayton State University) with the passion in mind to study Drama Therapy.

"Helping others heal is my life's work, I was created to facilitate a safe space for the growth and development of those in need."

- Maya C. Houston-

Mentor and Activist
South Carolina Notary Public
Published Author 2010
Publisher & Playwright
Spoken word & performance artist
Clayton State University graduate 2013 (B.A.)
Ohio Christian University Graduate 2023 (M.B.A.)

Facebook: @Maya C. Houston

Instagram: @minnamaya1

Symptoms & Causes

Symptoms:

All anxiety disorders share some general symptoms:
- Panic, fear, and uneasiness
- Sleep problems
- Not being able to stay calm and still
- Cold, sweaty, numb or tingling hands or feet
- Shortness of breath
- Heart palpitations
- Dry mouth
- Nausea
- Tense muscles
- Dizziness

Causes:

Researchers don't know exactly what brings on anxiety disorders. Like other forms of mental illness, they stem from a combination of things, including changes in your brain and environmental stress, and even your genes. The disorders can run in families and could be linked to faulty circuits in the brain that control fear and other emotions.

Hotlines

National Alliance on Mental Illness (NAMI)
1-800-950-NAMI(6264)

Anxiety and Addiction:
1-866-299-4557

National Suicide Prevention Lifeline
1-800-273-TALK(8255)

Substance Abuse and Mental Health Services Administration (SAMHSA)
1-800-662-HELP(4357)

Boys Town National Hotline
1-800-448-3000

Teen Line
1-800-TLC-TEEN(852-8336)